Color Me Groovy
1960'S
adult coloring book

ZenMaster Coloring Books

Helpful Tips for Coloring

~ Sometimes the colors appear differently on paper than what you would expect. Use the color test page to play with your colors beforehand.

~ If you are using colored pencils make sure to keep them sharp. This helps when coloring smaller areas or details on the page. Fine point sharpies also work great for smaller areas.

~ Speaking of sharpies, make sure you put a scrap piece of paper behind the page you are coloring to keep the markers from bleeding to the next page.

~ When using crayons or pencils start out light. You can always go back and darken later.

~ There are so many tools for coloring: markers, sharpies, crayons, pencils, pastels, and the list goes on. Experiment with what works best for you and your designs. Though it's not necessary, using higher quality coloring utensils makes a difference.

~ If you come to a design that seems overwhelming just pick a place to start and go from there. Once you begin your creativity will quickly take over!! If you get discouraged just take a break and come back to the page later.

~ Remember to practice. Like anything else, the more you do it the better you'll get. It'll become more and more relaxing each time.

~ DON'T FOLLOW THE RULES! It's up to you how you color your designs. Just let your creativity take the lead and HAVE FUN!

COLOR TEST PAGE

COLOR TEST PAGE

Thank you for supporting
ZenMaster Coloring Books

Your support means the world to us,
and we're thrilled to have you embark on this
creative journey with us.

Our small company strives to make a
BIG difference by helping those
who may be less fortunate.

This is why we proudly hire struggling
artists from around the world!

Our goal is to provide financial support to artists and
their families by enabling them to pursue their passions
and share their hard work and limitless talent with you!

Help support our hard working artists
by leaving a positive review on Amazon!

And follow us on Facebook for updates and
FREE COLORING PAGES!
https://www.facebook.com/zenmastercoloringbooks/

Check out more of our books at:
amazon.com/author/zenmastercoloringbooks

Free Bonus Page!
from:

Happy Summer
coloring book for adults

https://www.amazon.com/dp/1986950115

Also available in color by numbers!!
https://www.amazon.com/dp/1986983838

And a 5x8" Travel Size
https://www.amazon.com/dp/172614500X

Free Bonus Page!
from:

Guitars

Coloring Book for Men

https://amzn.com/dp/1545470855

Free Bonus Page!
from:

Extreme dot to dot book of
Butterflies and Flowers

https://amzn.com/dp/1717596746

Also available in color by numbers!!
https://www.amazon.com/dp/1977932398

And a non-numbered edition
https://www.amazon.com/dp/1977882978

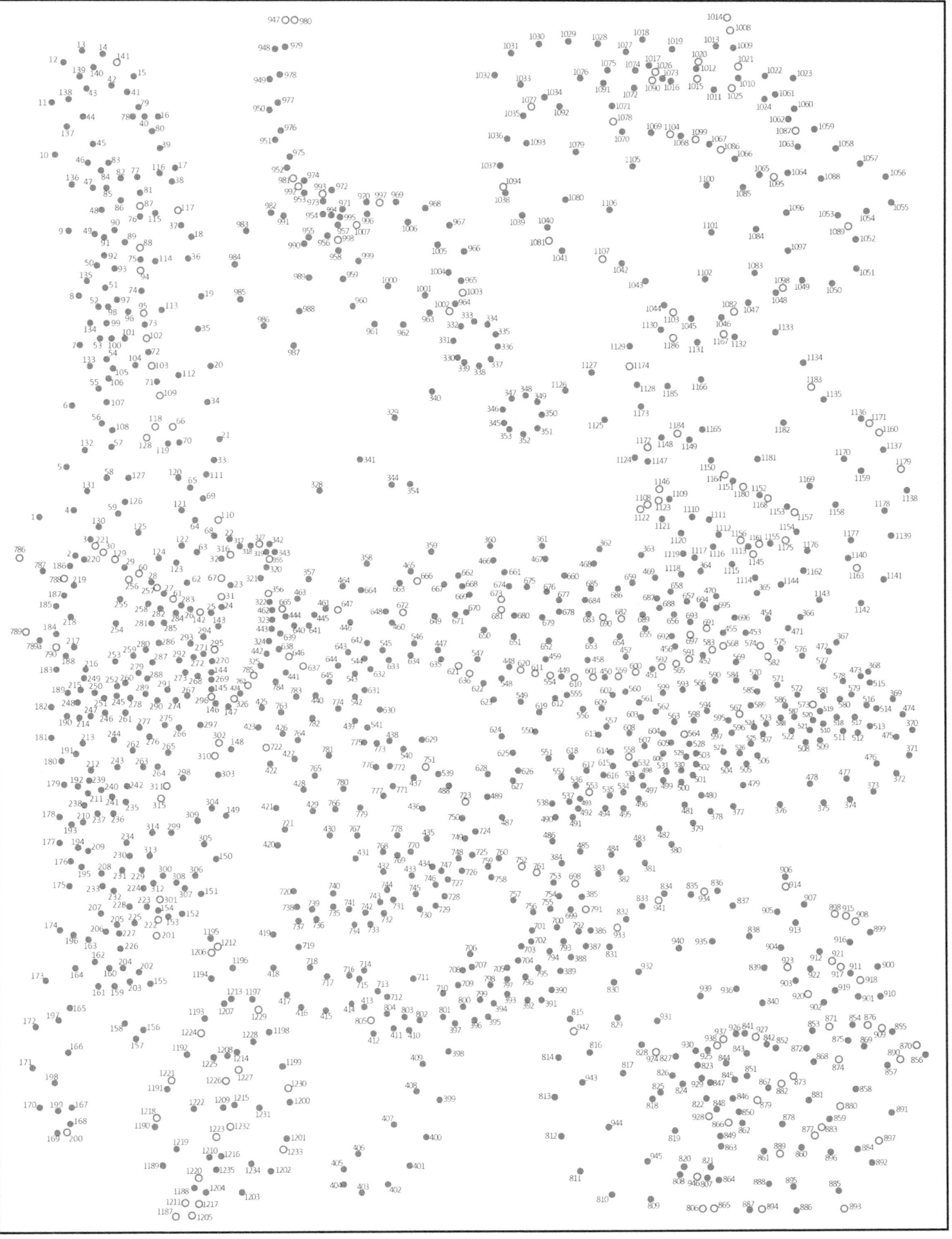

Free Bonus Page!
from:

Happy Hour
Adult Coloring Book

https://amzn.com/dp/1539662462

Also available in color by numbers!!
https://www.amazon.com/dp/1976119944

Free Bonus Page!
from:

Koi Fish
coloring book for adults

https://www.amazon.com/dp/1977939619

Also available in color by numbers!!
https://www.amazon.com/dp/198149104x

And 5x8" Travel Size
https://www.amazon.com/dp/1727375149

Free Bonus Page!
from:

Vogue 1950s
adult coloring book

https://www.amazon.com/dp/1973981521

Also available in color by numbers!!
https://www.amazon.com/dp/1978343884

And 5x8" Travel Size
https://www.amazon.com/dp/1973981610

Free Bonus Page!
from:

Zen Coloring Notebook

https://www.amazon.com/dp/1535457015

Available in 9 different colors!

Also available in 5x8" journal size
https://www.amazon.com/dp/1535540591

www.ingramcontent.com/pod-product-compliance
Lightning Source LLC
Chambersburg PA
CBHW081419280526
45788CB00009B/3158